WORKOUT LOG

NAME:________________________   GOALS:________________________

EXERCISES	SETS	REPS	WT	REST	TIME	1 RM	NOTES

DATE:_________   WEIGHT:_________   SLEEP:_________   CALORIES:_________

EXERCISES	SETS	REPS	WT	REST	TIME	1 RM	NOTES

DATE:_________   WEIGHT:_________   SLEEP:_________   CALORIES:_________

EXERCISES	SETS	REPS	WT	REST	TIME	1 RM	NOTES

DATE:_________   WEIGHT:_________   SLEEP:_________   CALORIES:_________

EXERCISES	SETS	REPS	WT	REST	TIME	1 RM	NOTES

DATE:_________   WEIGHT:_________   SLEEP:_________   CALORIES:_________

EXERCISES	SETS	REPS	WT	REST	TIME	1 RM	NOTES

DATE:_________   WEIGHT:_________   SLEEP:_________   CALORIES:_________

WORKOUT LOG

NAME:_________________________   GOALS:___________________________

EXERCISES	SETS	REPS	WT	REST	TIME	1 RM	NOTES

DATE:__________   WEIGHT:__________   SLEEP:__________   CALORIES:__________

EXERCISES	SETS	REPS	WT	REST	TIME	1 RM	NOTES

DATE:__________   WEIGHT:__________   SLEEP:__________   CALORIES:__________

EXERCISES	SETS	REPS	WT	REST	TIME	1 RM	NOTES

DATE:__________   WEIGHT:__________   SLEEP:__________   CALORIES:__________

EXERCISES	SETS	REPS	WT	REST	TIME	1 RM	NOTES

DATE:__________   WEIGHT:__________   SLEEP:__________   CALORIES:__________

EXERCISES	SETS	REPS	WT	REST	TIME	1 RM	NOTES

DATE:__________   WEIGHT:__________   SLEEP:__________   CALORIES:__________

WORKOUT LOG

NAME:________________________ GOALS:________________________

EXERCISES	SETS	REPS	WT	REST	TIME	1 RM	NOTES

DATE:__________ WEIGHT:__________ SLEEP:__________ CALORIES:__________

EXERCISES	SETS	REPS	WT	REST	TIME	1 RM	NOTES

DATE:__________ WEIGHT:__________ SLEEP:__________ CALORIES:__________

EXERCISES	SETS	REPS	WT	REST	TIME	1 RM	NOTES

DATE:__________ WEIGHT:__________ SLEEP:__________ CALORIES:__________

EXERCISES	SETS	REPS	WT	REST	TIME	1 RM	NOTES

DATE:__________ WEIGHT:__________ SLEEP:__________ CALORIES:__________

EXERCISES	SETS	REPS	WT	REST	TIME	1 RM	NOTES

DATE:__________ WEIGHT:__________ SLEEP:__________ CALORIES:__________

WORKOUT LOG

NAME:______________________ GOALS:______________________

EXERCISES	SETS	REPS	WT	REST	TIME	1 RM	NOTES

DATE:__________ WEIGHT:__________ SLEEP:__________ CALORIES:__________

EXERCISES	SETS	REPS	WT	REST	TIME	1 RM	NOTES

DATE:__________ WEIGHT:__________ SLEEP:__________ CALORIES:__________

EXERCISES	SETS	REPS	WT	REST	TIME	1 RM	NOTES

DATE:__________ WEIGHT:__________ SLEEP:__________ CALORIES:__________

EXERCISES	SETS	REPS	WT	REST	TIME	1 RM	NOTES

DATE:__________ WEIGHT:__________ SLEEP:__________ CALORIES:__________

EXERCISES	SETS	REPS	WT	REST	TIME	1 RM	NOTES

DATE:__________ WEIGHT:__________ SLEEP:__________ CALORIES:__________

WORKOUT LOG

NAME:_________________________   GOALS:_________________________

EXERCISES	SETS	REPS	WT	REST	TIME	1 RM	NOTES

DATE:__________   WEIGHT:__________   SLEEP:__________   CALORIES:__________

EXERCISES	SETS	REPS	WT	REST	TIME	1 RM	NOTES

DATE:__________   WEIGHT:__________   SLEEP:__________   CALORIES:__________

EXERCISES	SETS	REPS	WT	REST	TIME	1 RM	NOTES

DATE:__________   WEIGHT:__________   SLEEP:__________   CALORIES:__________

EXERCISES	SETS	REPS	WT	REST	TIME	1 RM	NOTES

DATE:__________   WEIGHT:__________   SLEEP:__________   CALORIES:__________

EXERCISES	SETS	REPS	WT	REST	TIME	1 RM	NOTES

DATE:__________   WEIGHT:__________   SLEEP:__________   CALORIES:__________

WORKOUT LOG

NAME:____________________ GOALS:____________________

EXERCISES	SETS	REPS	WT	REST	TIME	1 RM	NOTES

DATE:__________ WEIGHT:__________ SLEEP:__________ CALORIES:__________

EXERCISES	SETS	REPS	WT	REST	TIME	1 RM	NOTES

DATE:__________ WEIGHT:__________ SLEEP:__________ CALORIES:__________

EXERCISES	SETS	REPS	WT	REST	TIME	1 RM	NOTES

DATE:__________ WEIGHT:__________ SLEEP:__________ CALORIES:__________

EXERCISES	SETS	REPS	WT	REST	TIME	1 RM	NOTES

DATE:__________ WEIGHT:__________ SLEEP:__________ CALORIES:__________

EXERCISES	SETS	REPS	WT	REST	TIME	1 RM	NOTES

DATE:__________ WEIGHT:__________ SLEEP:__________ CALORIES:__________

WORKOUT LOG

NAME:_____________________________ GOALS:_____________________________

EXERCISES	SETS	REPS	WT	REST	TIME	1 RM	NOTES

DATE:__________ WEIGHT:__________ SLEEP:__________ CALORIES:__________

EXERCISES	SETS	REPS	WT	REST	TIME	1 RM	NOTES

DATE:__________ WEIGHT:__________ SLEEP:__________ CALORIES:__________

EXERCISES	SETS	REPS	WT	REST	TIME	1 RM	NOTES

DATE:__________ WEIGHT:__________ SLEEP:__________ CALORIES:__________

EXERCISES	SETS	REPS	WT	REST	TIME	1 RM	NOTES

DATE:__________ WEIGHT:__________ SLEEP:__________ CALORIES:__________

EXERCISES	SETS	REPS	WT	REST	TIME	1 RM	NOTES

DATE:__________ WEIGHT:__________ SLEEP:__________ CALORIES:__________

WORKOUT LOG

NAME:__________________________   GOALS:__________________________

EXERCISES	SETS	REPS	WT	REST	TIME	1 RM	NOTES

DATE:__________   WEIGHT:__________   SLEEP:__________   CALORIES:__________

EXERCISES	SETS	REPS	WT	REST	TIME	1 RM	NOTES

DATE:__________   WEIGHT:__________   SLEEP:__________   CALORIES:__________

EXERCISES	SETS	REPS	WT	REST	TIME	1 RM	NOTES

DATE:__________   WEIGHT:__________   SLEEP:__________   CALORIES:__________

EXERCISES	SETS	REPS	WT	REST	TIME	1 RM	NOTES

DATE:__________   WEIGHT:__________   SLEEP:__________   CALORIES:__________

EXERCISES	SETS	REPS	WT	REST	TIME	1 RM	NOTES

DATE:__________   WEIGHT:__________   SLEEP:__________   CALORIES:__________

WORKOUT LOG

NAME:_____________________________   GOALS:_____________________________

EXERCISES	SETS	REPS	WT	REST	TIME	1 RM	NOTES

DATE:__________   WEIGHT:__________   SLEEP:__________   CALORIES:__________

EXERCISES	SETS	REPS	WT	REST	TIME	1 RM	NOTES

DATE:__________   WEIGHT:__________   SLEEP:__________   CALORIES:__________

EXERCISES	SETS	REPS	WT	REST	TIME	1 RM	NOTES

DATE:__________   WEIGHT:__________   SLEEP:__________   CALORIES:__________

EXERCISES	SETS	REPS	WT	REST	TIME	1 RM	NOTES

DATE:__________   WEIGHT:__________   SLEEP:__________   CALORIES:__________

EXERCISES	SETS	REPS	WT	REST	TIME	1 RM	NOTES

DATE:__________   WEIGHT:__________   SLEEP:__________   CALORIES:__________

WORKOUT LOG

NAME:________________________   GOALS:________________________

EXERCISES	SETS	REPS	WT	REST	TIME	1 RM	NOTES

DATE:__________   WEIGHT:__________   SLEEP:__________   CALORIES:__________

EXERCISES	SETS	REPS	WT	REST	TIME	1 RM	NOTES

DATE:__________   WEIGHT:__________   SLEEP:__________   CALORIES:__________

EXERCISES	SETS	REPS	WT	REST	TIME	1 RM	NOTES

DATE:__________   WEIGHT:__________   SLEEP:__________   CALORIES:__________

EXERCISES	SETS	REPS	WT	REST	TIME	1 RM	NOTES

DATE:__________   WEIGHT:__________   SLEEP:__________   CALORIES:__________

EXERCISES	SETS	REPS	WT	REST	TIME	1 RM	NOTES

DATE:__________   WEIGHT:__________   SLEEP:__________   CALORIES:__________

WORKOUT LOG

NAME: ___________________________   GOALS: ___________________________

EXERCISES	SETS	REPS	WT	REST	TIME	1 RM	NOTES

DATE: __________   WEIGHT: __________   SLEEP: __________   CALORIES: __________

EXERCISES	SETS	REPS	WT	REST	TIME	1 RM	NOTES

DATE: __________   WEIGHT: __________   SLEEP: __________   CALORIES: __________

EXERCISES	SETS	REPS	WT	REST	TIME	1 RM	NOTES

DATE: __________   WEIGHT: __________   SLEEP: __________   CALORIES: __________

EXERCISES	SETS	REPS	WT	REST	TIME	1 RM	NOTES

DATE: __________   WEIGHT: __________   SLEEP: __________   CALORIES: __________

EXERCISES	SETS	REPS	WT	REST	TIME	1 RM	NOTES

DATE: __________   WEIGHT: __________   SLEEP: __________   CALORIES: __________

WORKOUT LOG

NAME:________________________________   GOALS:________________________________

EXERCISES	SETS	REPS	WT	REST	TIME	1 RM	NOTES

DATE:___________   WEIGHT:___________   SLEEP:___________   CALORIES:___________

EXERCISES	SETS	REPS	WT	REST	TIME	1 RM	NOTES

DATE:___________   WEIGHT:___________   SLEEP:___________   CALORIES:___________

EXERCISES	SETS	REPS	WT	REST	TIME	1 RM	NOTES

DATE:___________   WEIGHT:___________   SLEEP:___________   CALORIES:___________

EXERCISES	SETS	REPS	WT	REST	TIME	1 RM	NOTES

DATE:___________   WEIGHT:___________   SLEEP:___________   CALORIES:___________

EXERCISES	SETS	REPS	WT	REST	TIME	1 RM	NOTES

DATE:___________   WEIGHT:___________   SLEEP:___________   CALORIES:___________

WORKOUT LOG

NAME:_________________________ GOALS:___________________________

EXERCISES	SETS	REPS	WT	REST	TIME	1 RM	NOTES

DATE:__________ WEIGHT:__________ SLEEP:__________ CALORIES:__________

EXERCISES	SETS	REPS	WT	REST	TIME	1 RM	NOTES

DATE:__________ WEIGHT:__________ SLEEP:__________ CALORIES:__________

EXERCISES	SETS	REPS	WT	REST	TIME	1 RM	NOTES

DATE:__________ WEIGHT:__________ SLEEP:__________ CALORIES:__________

EXERCISES	SETS	REPS	WT	REST	TIME	1 RM	NOTES

DATE:__________ WEIGHT:__________ SLEEP:__________ CALORIES:__________

EXERCISES	SETS	REPS	WT	REST	TIME	1 RM	NOTES

DATE:__________ WEIGHT:__________ SLEEP:__________ CALORIES:__________

WORKOUT LOG

NAME:__________________________ GOALS:__________________________

EXERCISES	SETS	REPS	WT	REST	TIME	1 RM	NOTES

DATE:__________ WEIGHT:__________ SLEEP:__________ CALORIES:__________

EXERCISES	SETS	REPS	WT	REST	TIME	1 RM	NOTES

DATE:__________ WEIGHT:__________ SLEEP:__________ CALORIES:__________

EXERCISES	SETS	REPS	WT	REST	TIME	1 RM	NOTES

DATE:__________ WEIGHT:__________ SLEEP:__________ CALORIES:__________

EXERCISES	SETS	REPS	WT	REST	TIME	1 RM	NOTES

DATE:__________ WEIGHT:__________ SLEEP:__________ CALORIES:__________

EXERCISES	SETS	REPS	WT	REST	TIME	1 RM	NOTES

DATE:__________ WEIGHT:__________ SLEEP:__________ CALORIES:__________

WORKOUT LOG

NAME:_________________________ GOALS:_____________________________

EXERCISES	SETS	REPS	WT	REST	TIME	1 RM	NOTES

DATE:__________ WEIGHT:__________ SLEEP:__________ CALORIES:__________

EXERCISES	SETS	REPS	WT	REST	TIME	1 RM	NOTES

DATE:__________ WEIGHT:__________ SLEEP:__________ CALORIES:__________

EXERCISES	SETS	REPS	WT	REST	TIME	1 RM	NOTES

DATE:__________ WEIGHT:__________ SLEEP:__________ CALORIES:__________

EXERCISES	SETS	REPS	WT	REST	TIME	1 RM	NOTES

DATE:__________ WEIGHT:__________ SLEEP:__________ CALORIES:__________

EXERCISES	SETS	REPS	WT	REST	TIME	1 RM	NOTES

DATE:__________ WEIGHT:__________ SLEEP:__________ CALORIES:__________

WORKOUT LOG

NAME:_______________________________ GOALS:_______________________________

EXERCISES	SETS	REPS	WT	REST	TIME	1 RM	NOTES

DATE:__________   WEIGHT:__________   SLEEP:__________   CALORIES:__________

EXERCISES	SETS	REPS	WT	REST	TIME	1 RM	NOTES

DATE:__________   WEIGHT:__________   SLEEP:__________   CALORIES:__________

EXERCISES	SETS	REPS	WT	REST	TIME	1 RM	NOTES

DATE:__________   WEIGHT:__________   SLEEP:__________   CALORIES:__________

EXERCISES	SETS	REPS	WT	REST	TIME	1 RM	NOTES

DATE:__________   WEIGHT:__________   SLEEP:__________   CALORIES:__________

EXERCISES	SETS	REPS	WT	REST	TIME	1 RM	NOTES

DATE:__________   WEIGHT:__________   SLEEP:__________   CALORIES:__________

WORKOUT LOG

NAME:_________________________ GOALS:_________________________

EXERCISES	SETS	REPS	WT	REST	TIME	1 RM	NOTES

DATE:__________ WEIGHT:__________ SLEEP:__________ CALORIES:__________

EXERCISES	SETS	REPS	WT	REST	TIME	1 RM	NOTES

DATE:__________ WEIGHT:__________ SLEEP:__________ CALORIES:__________

EXERCISES	SETS	REPS	WT	REST	TIME	1 RM	NOTES

DATE:__________ WEIGHT:__________ SLEEP:__________ CALORIES:__________

EXERCISES	SETS	REPS	WT	REST	TIME	1 RM	NOTES

DATE:__________ WEIGHT:__________ SLEEP:__________ CALORIES:__________

EXERCISES	SETS	REPS	WT	REST	TIME	1 RM	NOTES

DATE:__________ WEIGHT:__________ SLEEP:__________ CALORIES:__________

WORKOUT LOG

NAME:________________________ GOALS:__________________________

EXERCISES	SETS	REPS	WT	REST	TIME	1 RM	NOTES

DATE:__________   WEIGHT:__________   SLEEP:__________   CALORIES:__________

EXERCISES	SETS	REPS	WT	REST	TIME	1 RM	NOTES

DATE:__________   WEIGHT:__________   SLEEP:__________   CALORIES:__________

EXERCISES	SETS	REPS	WT	REST	TIME	1 RM	NOTES

DATE:__________   WEIGHT:__________   SLEEP:__________   CALORIES:__________

EXERCISES	SETS	REPS	WT	REST	TIME	1 RM	NOTES

DATE:__________   WEIGHT:__________   SLEEP:__________   CALORIES:__________

EXERCISES	SETS	REPS	WT	REST	TIME	1 RM	NOTES

DATE:__________   WEIGHT:__________   SLEEP:__________   CALORIES:__________

WORKOUT LOG

NAME:_______________________ GOALS:_______________________

EXERCISES	SETS	REPS	WT	REST	TIME	1 RM	NOTES

DATE:__________ WEIGHT:__________ SLEEP:__________ CALORIES:__________

EXERCISES	SETS	REPS	WT	REST	TIME	1 RM	NOTES

DATE:__________ WEIGHT:__________ SLEEP:__________ CALORIES:__________

EXERCISES	SETS	REPS	WT	REST	TIME	1 RM	NOTES

DATE:__________ WEIGHT:__________ SLEEP:__________ CALORIES:__________

EXERCISES	SETS	REPS	WT	REST	TIME	1 RM	NOTES

DATE:__________ WEIGHT:__________ SLEEP:__________ CALORIES:__________

EXERCISES	SETS	REPS	WT	REST	TIME	1 RM	NOTES

DATE:__________ WEIGHT:__________ SLEEP:__________ CALORIES:__________

WORKOUT LOG

NAME:_________________________ GOALS:_________________________

EXERCISES	SETS	REPS	WT	REST	TIME	1 RM	NOTES

DATE:__________ WEIGHT:__________ SLEEP:__________ CALORIES:__________

EXERCISES	SETS	REPS	WT	REST	TIME	1 RM	NOTES

DATE:__________ WEIGHT:__________ SLEEP:__________ CALORIES:__________

EXERCISES	SETS	REPS	WT	REST	TIME	1 RM	NOTES

DATE:__________ WEIGHT:__________ SLEEP:__________ CALORIES:__________

EXERCISES	SETS	REPS	WT	REST	TIME	1 RM	NOTES

DATE:__________ WEIGHT:__________ SLEEP:__________ CALORIES:__________

EXERCISES	SETS	REPS	WT	REST	TIME	1 RM	NOTES

DATE:__________ WEIGHT:__________ SLEEP:__________ CALORIES:__________

WORKOUT LOG

NAME:_______________________   GOALS:_______________________

EXERCISES	SETS	REPS	WT	REST	TIME	1 RM	NOTES

DATE:__________   WEIGHT:__________   SLEEP:__________   CALORIES:__________

EXERCISES	SETS	REPS	WT	REST	TIME	1 RM	NOTES

DATE:__________   WEIGHT:__________   SLEEP:__________   CALORIES:__________

EXERCISES	SETS	REPS	WT	REST	TIME	1 RM	NOTES

DATE:__________   WEIGHT:__________   SLEEP:__________   CALORIES:__________

EXERCISES	SETS	REPS	WT	REST	TIME	1 RM	NOTES

DATE:__________   WEIGHT:__________   SLEEP:__________   CALORIES:__________

EXERCISES	SETS	REPS	WT	REST	TIME	1 RM	NOTES

DATE:__________   WEIGHT:__________   SLEEP:__________   CALORIES:__________

WORKOUT LOG

NAME:________________________ GOALS:________________________

EXERCISES	SETS	REPS	WT	REST	TIME	1 RM	NOTES

DATE:________ WEIGHT:________ SLEEP:________ CALORIES:________

EXERCISES	SETS	REPS	WT	REST	TIME	1 RM	NOTES

DATE:________ WEIGHT:________ SLEEP:________ CALORIES:________

EXERCISES	SETS	REPS	WT	REST	TIME	1 RM	NOTES

DATE:________ WEIGHT:________ SLEEP:________ CALORIES:________

EXERCISES	SETS	REPS	WT	REST	TIME	1 RM	NOTES

DATE:________ WEIGHT:________ SLEEP:________ CALORIES:________

EXERCISES	SETS	REPS	WT	REST	TIME	1 RM	NOTES

DATE:________ WEIGHT:________ SLEEP:________ CALORIES:________

WORKOUT LOG

NAME:________________________   GOALS:________________________

EXERCISES	SETS	REPS	WT	REST	TIME	1 RM	NOTES

DATE:__________   WEIGHT:__________   SLEEP:__________   CALORIES:__________

EXERCISES	SETS	REPS	WT	REST	TIME	1 RM	NOTES

DATE:__________   WEIGHT:__________   SLEEP:__________   CALORIES:__________

EXERCISES	SETS	REPS	WT	REST	TIME	1 RM	NOTES

DATE:__________   WEIGHT:__________   SLEEP:__________   CALORIES:__________

EXERCISES	SETS	REPS	WT	REST	TIME	1 RM	NOTES

DATE:__________   WEIGHT:__________   SLEEP:__________   CALORIES:__________

EXERCISES	SETS	REPS	WT	REST	TIME	1 RM	NOTES

DATE:__________   WEIGHT:__________   SLEEP:__________   CALORIES:__________

WORKOUT LOG

NAME: _________________________ GOALS: _________________________

EXERCISES	SETS	REPS	WT	REST	TIME	1 RM	NOTES

DATE: __________ WEIGHT: __________ SLEEP: __________ CALORIES: __________

EXERCISES	SETS	REPS	WT	REST	TIME	1 RM	NOTES

DATE: __________ WEIGHT: __________ SLEEP: __________ CALORIES: __________

EXERCISES	SETS	REPS	WT	REST	TIME	1 RM	NOTES

DATE: __________ WEIGHT: __________ SLEEP: __________ CALORIES: __________

EXERCISES	SETS	REPS	WT	REST	TIME	1 RM	NOTES

DATE: __________ WEIGHT: __________ SLEEP: __________ CALORIES: __________

EXERCISES	SETS	REPS	WT	REST	TIME	1 RM	NOTES

DATE: __________ WEIGHT: __________ SLEEP: __________ CALORIES: __________

WORKOUT LOG

NAME:_________________________ GOALS:___________________________

EXERCISES	SETS	REPS	WT	REST	TIME	1 RM	NOTES

DATE:__________   WEIGHT:__________   SLEEP:__________   CALORIES:__________

EXERCISES	SETS	REPS	WT	REST	TIME	1 RM	NOTES

DATE:__________   WEIGHT:__________   SLEEP:__________   CALORIES:__________

EXERCISES	SETS	REPS	WT	REST	TIME	1 RM	NOTES

DATE:__________   WEIGHT:__________   SLEEP:__________   CALORIES:__________

EXERCISES	SETS	REPS	WT	REST	TIME	1 RM	NOTES

DATE:__________   WEIGHT:__________   SLEEP:__________   CALORIES:__________

EXERCISES	SETS	REPS	WT	REST	TIME	1 RM	NOTES

DATE:__________   WEIGHT:__________   SLEEP:__________   CALORIES:__________

WORKOUT LOG

NAME:________________________ GOALS:________________________

EXERCISES	SETS	REPS	WT	REST	TIME	1 RM	NOTES

DATE:__________ WEIGHT:__________ SLEEP:__________ CALORIES:__________

EXERCISES	SETS	REPS	WT	REST	TIME	1 RM	NOTES

DATE:__________ WEIGHT:__________ SLEEP:__________ CALORIES:__________

EXERCISES	SETS	REPS	WT	REST	TIME	1 RM	NOTES

DATE:__________ WEIGHT:__________ SLEEP:__________ CALORIES:__________

EXERCISES	SETS	REPS	WT	REST	TIME	1 RM	NOTES

DATE:__________ WEIGHT:__________ SLEEP:__________ CALORIES:__________

EXERCISES	SETS	REPS	WT	REST	TIME	1 RM	NOTES

DATE:__________ WEIGHT:__________ SLEEP:__________ CALORIES:__________

WORKOUT LOG

NAME:__________________________   GOALS:__________________________

EXERCISES	SETS	REPS	WT	REST	TIME	1 RM	NOTES

DATE:__________   WEIGHT:__________   SLEEP:__________   CALORIES:__________

EXERCISES	SETS	REPS	WT	REST	TIME	1 RM	NOTES

DATE:__________   WEIGHT:__________   SLEEP:__________   CALORIES:__________

EXERCISES	SETS	REPS	WT	REST	TIME	1 RM	NOTES

DATE:__________   WEIGHT:__________   SLEEP:__________   CALORIES:__________

EXERCISES	SETS	REPS	WT	REST	TIME	1 RM	NOTES

DATE:__________   WEIGHT:__________   SLEEP:__________   CALORIES:__________

EXERCISES	SETS	REPS	WT	REST	TIME	1 RM	NOTES

DATE:__________   WEIGHT:__________   SLEEP:__________   CALORIES:__________

WORKOUT LOG

NAME:_____________________________ GOALS:_____________________________

EXERCISES	SETS	REPS	WT	REST	TIME	1 RM	NOTES

DATE:__________ WEIGHT:__________ SLEEP:__________ CALORIES:__________

EXERCISES	SETS	REPS	WT	REST	TIME	1 RM	NOTES

DATE:__________ WEIGHT:__________ SLEEP:__________ CALORIES:__________

EXERCISES	SETS	REPS	WT	REST	TIME	1 RM	NOTES

DATE:__________ WEIGHT:__________ SLEEP:__________ CALORIES:__________

EXERCISES	SETS	REPS	WT	REST	TIME	1 RM	NOTES

DATE:__________ WEIGHT:__________ SLEEP:__________ CALORIES:__________

EXERCISES	SETS	REPS	WT	REST	TIME	1 RM	NOTES

DATE:__________ WEIGHT:__________ SLEEP:__________ CALORIES:__________

WORKOUT LOG

NAME:_________________________   GOALS:_____________________

EXERCISES	SETS	REPS	WT	REST	TIME	1 RM	NOTES

DATE:__________   WEIGHT:__________   SLEEP:__________   CALORIES:__________

EXERCISES	SETS	REPS	WT	REST	TIME	1 RM	NOTES

DATE:__________   WEIGHT:__________   SLEEP:__________   CALORIES:__________

EXERCISES	SETS	REPS	WT	REST	TIME	1 RM	NOTES

DATE:__________   WEIGHT:__________   SLEEP:__________   CALORIES:__________

EXERCISES	SETS	REPS	WT	REST	TIME	1 RM	NOTES

DATE:__________   WEIGHT:__________   SLEEP:__________   CALORIES:__________

EXERCISES	SETS	REPS	WT	REST	TIME	1 RM	NOTES

DATE:__________   WEIGHT:__________   SLEEP:__________   CALORIES:__________

WORKOUT LOG

NAME:_________________________ GOALS:___________________________

EXERCISES	SETS	REPS	WT	REST	TIME	1 RM	NOTES

DATE:__________ WEIGHT:__________ SLEEP:__________ CALORIES:__________

EXERCISES	SETS	REPS	WT	REST	TIME	1 RM	NOTES

DATE:__________ WEIGHT:__________ SLEEP:__________ CALORIES:__________

EXERCISES	SETS	REPS	WT	REST	TIME	1 RM	NOTES

DATE:__________ WEIGHT:__________ SLEEP:__________ CALORIES:__________

EXERCISES	SETS	REPS	WT	REST	TIME	1 RM	NOTES

DATE:__________ WEIGHT:__________ SLEEP:__________ CALORIES:__________

EXERCISES	SETS	REPS	WT	REST	TIME	1 RM	NOTES

DATE:__________ WEIGHT:__________ SLEEP:__________ CALORIES:__________

WORKOUT LOG

NAME:_______________________   GOALS:_____________________

EXERCISES	SETS	REPS	WT	REST	TIME	1RM	NOTES

DATE:_________   WEIGHT:_________   SLEEP:_________   CALORIES:_________

EXERCISES	SETS	REPS	WT	REST	TIME	1RM	NOTES

DATE:_________   WEIGHT:_________   SLEEP:_________   CALORIES:_________

EXERCISES	SETS	REPS	WT	REST	TIME	1RM	NOTES

DATE:_________   WEIGHT:_________   SLEEP:_________   CALORIES:_________

EXERCISES	SETS	REPS	WT	REST	TIME	1RM	NOTES

DATE:_________   WEIGHT:_________   SLEEP:_________   CALORIES:_________

EXERCISES	SETS	REPS	WT	REST	TIME	1RM	NOTES

DATE:_________   WEIGHT:_________   SLEEP:_________   CALORIES:_________

WORKOUT LOG

NAME:________________________ GOALS:________________________

EXERCISES	SETS	REPS	WT	REST	TIME	1 RM	NOTES

DATE:__________ WEIGHT:__________ SLEEP:__________ CALORIES:__________

EXERCISES	SETS	REPS	WT	REST	TIME	1 RM	NOTES

DATE:__________ WEIGHT:__________ SLEEP:__________ CALORIES:__________

EXERCISES	SETS	REPS	WT	REST	TIME	1 RM	NOTES

DATE:__________ WEIGHT:__________ SLEEP:__________ CALORIES:__________

EXERCISES	SETS	REPS	WT	REST	TIME	1 RM	NOTES

DATE:__________ WEIGHT:__________ SLEEP:__________ CALORIES:__________

EXERCISES	SETS	REPS	WT	REST	TIME	1 RM	NOTES

DATE:__________ WEIGHT:__________ SLEEP:__________ CALORIES:__________

WORKOUT LOG

NAME:_________________________   GOALS:_______________________

EXERCISES	SETS	REPS	WT	REST	TIME	1 RM	NOTES

DATE:__________   WEIGHT:__________   SLEEP:__________   CALORIES:__________

EXERCISES	SETS	REPS	WT	REST	TIME	1 RM	NOTES

DATE:__________   WEIGHT:__________   SLEEP:__________   CALORIES:__________

EXERCISES	SETS	REPS	WT	REST	TIME	1 RM	NOTES

DATE:__________   WEIGHT:__________   SLEEP:__________   CALORIES:__________

EXERCISES	SETS	REPS	WT	REST	TIME	1 RM	NOTES

DATE:__________   WEIGHT:__________   SLEEP:__________   CALORIES:__________

EXERCISES	SETS	REPS	WT	REST	TIME	1 RM	NOTES

DATE:__________   WEIGHT:__________   SLEEP:__________   CALORIES:__________

WORKOUT LOG

NAME:____________________________   GOALS:____________________________

EXERCISES	SETS	REPS	WT	REST	TIME	1 RM	NOTES

DATE:__________   WEIGHT:__________   SLEEP:__________   CALORIES:__________

EXERCISES	SETS	REPS	WT	REST	TIME	1 RM	NOTES

DATE:__________   WEIGHT:__________   SLEEP:__________   CALORIES:__________

EXERCISES	SETS	REPS	WT	REST	TIME	1 RM	NOTES

DATE:__________   WEIGHT:__________   SLEEP:__________   CALORIES:__________

EXERCISES	SETS	REPS	WT	REST	TIME	1 RM	NOTES

DATE:__________   WEIGHT:__________   SLEEP:__________   CALORIES:__________

EXERCISES	SETS	REPS	WT	REST	TIME	1 RM	NOTES

DATE:__________   WEIGHT:__________   SLEEP:__________   CALORIES:__________

WORKOUT LOG

NAME:_________________________   GOALS:_____________________

EXERCISES	SETS	REPS	WT	REST	TIME	1 RM	NOTES

DATE:__________   WEIGHT:__________   SLEEP:__________   CALORIES:__________

EXERCISES	SETS	REPS	WT	REST	TIME	1 RM	NOTES

DATE:__________   WEIGHT:__________   SLEEP:__________   CALORIES:__________

EXERCISES	SETS	REPS	WT	REST	TIME	1 RM	NOTES

DATE:__________   WEIGHT:__________   SLEEP:__________   CALORIES:__________

EXERCISES	SETS	REPS	WT	REST	TIME	1 RM	NOTES

DATE:__________   WEIGHT:__________   SLEEP:__________   CALORIES:__________

EXERCISES	SETS	REPS	WT	REST	TIME	1 RM	NOTES

DATE:__________   WEIGHT:__________   SLEEP:__________   CALORIES:__________

WORKOUT LOG

NAME:_____________________ GOALS:_____________________

EXERCISES	SETS	REPS	WT	REST	TIME	1 RM	NOTES

DATE:__________ WEIGHT:__________ SLEEP:__________ CALORIES:__________

EXERCISES	SETS	REPS	WT	REST	TIME	1 RM	NOTES

DATE:__________ WEIGHT:__________ SLEEP:__________ CALORIES:__________

EXERCISES	SETS	REPS	WT	REST	TIME	1 RM	NOTES

DATE:__________ WEIGHT:__________ SLEEP:__________ CALORIES:__________

EXERCISES	SETS	REPS	WT	REST	TIME	1 RM	NOTES

DATE:__________ WEIGHT:__________ SLEEP:__________ CALORIES:__________

EXERCISES	SETS	REPS	WT	REST	TIME	1 RM	NOTES

DATE:__________ WEIGHT:__________ SLEEP:__________ CALORIES:__________

WORKOUT LOG

NAME:_________________________ GOALS:_____________________

EXERCISES	SETS	REPS	WT	REST	TIME	1RM	NOTES

DATE:_________ WEIGHT:_________ SLEEP:_________ CALORIES:_________

EXERCISES	SETS	REPS	WT	REST	TIME	1RM	NOTES

DATE:_________ WEIGHT:_________ SLEEP:_________ CALORIES:_________

EXERCISES	SETS	REPS	WT	REST	TIME	1RM	NOTES

DATE:_________ WEIGHT:_________ SLEEP:_________ CALORIES:_________

EXERCISES	SETS	REPS	WT	REST	TIME	1RM	NOTES

DATE:_________ WEIGHT:_________ SLEEP:_________ CALORIES:_________

EXERCISES	SETS	REPS	WT	REST	TIME	1RM	NOTES

DATE:_________ WEIGHT:_________ SLEEP:_________ CALORIES:_________

WORKOUT LOG

NAME:_________________________ GOALS:_____________________________

EXERCISES	SETS	REPS	WT	REST	TIME	1 RM	NOTES

DATE:__________ WEIGHT:__________ SLEEP:__________ CALORIES:__________

EXERCISES	SETS	REPS	WT	REST	TIME	1 RM	NOTES

DATE:__________ WEIGHT:__________ SLEEP:__________ CALORIES:__________

EXERCISES	SETS	REPS	WT	REST	TIME	1 RM	NOTES

DATE:__________ WEIGHT:__________ SLEEP:__________ CALORIES:__________

EXERCISES	SETS	REPS	WT	REST	TIME	1 RM	NOTES

DATE:__________ WEIGHT:__________ SLEEP:__________ CALORIES:__________

EXERCISES	SETS	REPS	WT	REST	TIME	1 RM	NOTES

DATE:__________ WEIGHT:__________ SLEEP:__________ CALORIES:__________

WORKOUT LOG

NAME:__________________________   GOALS:__________________________

EXERCISES	SETS	REPS	WT	REST	TIME	1 RM	NOTES

DATE:__________   WEIGHT:__________   SLEEP:__________   CALORIES:__________

EXERCISES	SETS	REPS	WT	REST	TIME	1 RM	NOTES

DATE:__________   WEIGHT:__________   SLEEP:__________   CALORIES:__________

EXERCISES	SETS	REPS	WT	REST	TIME	1 RM	NOTES

DATE:__________   WEIGHT:__________   SLEEP:__________   CALORIES:__________

EXERCISES	SETS	REPS	WT	REST	TIME	1 RM	NOTES

DATE:__________   WEIGHT:__________   SLEEP:__________   CALORIES:__________

EXERCISES	SETS	REPS	WT	REST	TIME	1 RM	NOTES

DATE:__________   WEIGHT:__________   SLEEP:__________   CALORIES:__________

WORKOUT LOG

NAME:________________________   GOALS:__________________________

EXERCISES	SETS	REPS	WT	REST	TIME	1 RM	NOTES

DATE:__________   WEIGHT:__________   SLEEP:__________   CALORIES:__________

EXERCISES	SETS	REPS	WT	REST	TIME	1 RM	NOTES

DATE:__________   WEIGHT:__________   SLEEP:__________   CALORIES:__________

EXERCISES	SETS	REPS	WT	REST	TIME	1 RM	NOTES

DATE:__________   WEIGHT:__________   SLEEP:__________   CALORIES:__________

EXERCISES	SETS	REPS	WT	REST	TIME	1 RM	NOTES

DATE:__________   WEIGHT:__________   SLEEP:__________   CALORIES:__________

EXERCISES	SETS	REPS	WT	REST	TIME	1 RM	NOTES

DATE:__________   WEIGHT:__________   SLEEP:__________   CALORIES:__________

WORKOUT LOG

NAME:______________________________ GOALS:______________________________

EXERCISES	SETS	REPS	WT	REST	TIME	1 RM	NOTES

DATE:__________ WEIGHT:__________ SLEEP:__________ CALORIES:__________

EXERCISES	SETS	REPS	WT	REST	TIME	1 RM	NOTES

DATE:__________ WEIGHT:__________ SLEEP:__________ CALORIES:__________

EXERCISES	SETS	REPS	WT	REST	TIME	1 RM	NOTES

DATE:__________ WEIGHT:__________ SLEEP:__________ CALORIES:__________

EXERCISES	SETS	REPS	WT	REST	TIME	1 RM	NOTES

DATE:__________ WEIGHT:__________ SLEEP:__________ CALORIES:__________

EXERCISES	SETS	REPS	WT	REST	TIME	1 RM	NOTES

DATE:__________ WEIGHT:__________ SLEEP:__________ CALORIES:__________

WORKOUT LOG

NAME:_______________________ GOALS:_______________________

EXERCISES	SETS	REPS	WT	REST	TIME	1 RM	NOTES

DATE:__________ WEIGHT:__________ SLEEP:__________ CALORIES:__________

EXERCISES	SETS	REPS	WT	REST	TIME	1 RM	NOTES

DATE:__________ WEIGHT:__________ SLEEP:__________ CALORIES:__________

EXERCISES	SETS	REPS	WT	REST	TIME	1 RM	NOTES

DATE:__________ WEIGHT:__________ SLEEP:__________ CALORIES:__________

EXERCISES	SETS	REPS	WT	REST	TIME	1 RM	NOTES

DATE:__________ WEIGHT:__________ SLEEP:__________ CALORIES:__________

EXERCISES	SETS	REPS	WT	REST	TIME	1 RM	NOTES

DATE:__________ WEIGHT:__________ SLEEP:__________ CALORIES:__________

WORKOUT LOG

NAME:_______________________ GOALS:_______________________

EXERCISES	SETS	REPS	WT	REST	TIME	1 RM	NOTES

DATE:__________ WEIGHT:__________ SLEEP:__________ CALORIES:__________

EXERCISES	SETS	REPS	WT	REST	TIME	1 RM	NOTES

DATE:__________ WEIGHT:__________ SLEEP:__________ CALORIES:__________

EXERCISES	SETS	REPS	WT	REST	TIME	1 RM	NOTES

DATE:__________ WEIGHT:__________ SLEEP:__________ CALORIES:__________

EXERCISES	SETS	REPS	WT	REST	TIME	1 RM	NOTES

DATE:__________ WEIGHT:__________ SLEEP:__________ CALORIES:__________

EXERCISES	SETS	REPS	WT	REST	TIME	1 RM	NOTES

DATE:__________ WEIGHT:__________ SLEEP:__________ CALORIES:__________

WORKOUT LOG

NAME:_________________________ GOALS:_____________________

EXERCISES	SETS	REPS	WT	REST	TIME	1 RM	NOTES

DATE:__________ WEIGHT:__________ SLEEP:__________ CALORIES:__________

EXERCISES	SETS	REPS	WT	REST	TIME	1 RM	NOTES

DATE:__________ WEIGHT:__________ SLEEP:__________ CALORIES:__________

EXERCISES	SETS	REPS	WT	REST	TIME	1 RM	NOTES

DATE:__________ WEIGHT:__________ SLEEP:__________ CALORIES:__________

EXERCISES	SETS	REPS	WT	REST	TIME	1 RM	NOTES

DATE:__________ WEIGHT:__________ SLEEP:__________ CALORIES:__________

EXERCISES	SETS	REPS	WT	REST	TIME	1 RM	NOTES

DATE:__________ WEIGHT:__________ SLEEP:__________ CALORIES:__________

WORKOUT LOG

NAME:________________________ GOALS:________________________

EXERCISES	SETS	REPS	WT	REST	TIME	1 RM	NOTES

DATE:__________ WEIGHT:__________ SLEEP:__________ CALORIES:__________

EXERCISES	SETS	REPS	WT	REST	TIME	1 RM	NOTES

DATE:__________ WEIGHT:__________ SLEEP:__________ CALORIES:__________

EXERCISES	SETS	REPS	WT	REST	TIME	1 RM	NOTES

DATE:__________ WEIGHT:__________ SLEEP:__________ CALORIES:__________

EXERCISES	SETS	REPS	WT	REST	TIME	1 RM	NOTES

DATE:__________ WEIGHT:__________ SLEEP:__________ CALORIES:__________

EXERCISES	SETS	REPS	WT	REST	TIME	1 RM	NOTES

DATE:__________ WEIGHT:__________ SLEEP:__________ CALORIES:__________

WORKOUT LOG

NAME:_____________________________ GOALS:___________________________

EXERCISES	SETS	REPS	WT	REST	TIME	1 RM	NOTES

DATE:__________ WEIGHT:__________ SLEEP:__________ CALORIES:__________

EXERCISES	SETS	REPS	WT	REST	TIME	1 RM	NOTES

DATE:__________ WEIGHT:__________ SLEEP:__________ CALORIES:__________

EXERCISES	SETS	REPS	WT	REST	TIME	1 RM	NOTES

DATE:__________ WEIGHT:__________ SLEEP:__________ CALORIES:__________

EXERCISES	SETS	REPS	WT	REST	TIME	1 RM	NOTES

DATE:__________ WEIGHT:__________ SLEEP:__________ CALORIES:__________

EXERCISES	SETS	REPS	WT	REST	TIME	1 RM	NOTES

DATE:__________ WEIGHT:__________ SLEEP:__________ CALORIES:__________

WORKOUT LOG

NAME:___________________________ GOALS:____________________________

EXERCISES	SETS	REPS	WT	REST	TIME	1 RM	NOTES

DATE:__________   WEIGHT:__________   SLEEP:__________   CALORIES:__________

EXERCISES	SETS	REPS	WT	REST	TIME	1 RM	NOTES

DATE:__________   WEIGHT:__________   SLEEP:__________   CALORIES:__________

EXERCISES	SETS	REPS	WT	REST	TIME	1 RM	NOTES

DATE:__________   WEIGHT:__________   SLEEP:__________   CALORIES:__________

EXERCISES	SETS	REPS	WT	REST	TIME	1 RM	NOTES

DATE:__________   WEIGHT:__________   SLEEP:__________   CALORIES:__________

EXERCISES	SETS	REPS	WT	REST	TIME	1 RM	NOTES

DATE:__________   WEIGHT:__________   SLEEP:__________   CALORIES:__________

WORKOUT LOG

NAME:_________________________ GOALS:_________________________

EXERCISES	SETS	REPS	WT	REST	TIME	1 RM	NOTES

DATE:__________   WEIGHT:__________   SLEEP:__________   CALORIES:__________

EXERCISES	SETS	REPS	WT	REST	TIME	1 RM	NOTES

DATE:__________   WEIGHT:__________   SLEEP:__________   CALORIES:__________

EXERCISES	SETS	REPS	WT	REST	TIME	1 RM	NOTES

DATE:__________   WEIGHT:__________   SLEEP:__________   CALORIES:__________

EXERCISES	SETS	REPS	WT	REST	TIME	1 RM	NOTES

DATE:__________   WEIGHT:__________   SLEEP:__________   CALORIES:__________

EXERCISES	SETS	REPS	WT	REST	TIME	1 RM	NOTES

DATE:__________   WEIGHT:__________   SLEEP:__________   CALORIES:__________

WORKOUT LOG

NAME:_________________________ GOALS:_________________________

EXERCISES	SETS	REPS	WT	REST	TIME	1 RM	NOTES

DATE:_________ WEIGHT:_________ SLEEP:_________ CALORIES:_________

EXERCISES	SETS	REPS	WT	REST	TIME	1 RM	NOTES

DATE:_________ WEIGHT:_________ SLEEP:_________ CALORIES:_________

EXERCISES	SETS	REPS	WT	REST	TIME	1 RM	NOTES

DATE:_________ WEIGHT:_________ SLEEP:_________ CALORIES:_________

EXERCISES	SETS	REPS	WT	REST	TIME	1 RM	NOTES

DATE:_________ WEIGHT:_________ SLEEP:_________ CALORIES:_________

EXERCISES	SETS	REPS	WT	REST	TIME	1 RM	NOTES

DATE:_________ WEIGHT:_________ SLEEP:_________ CALORIES:_________

WORKOUT LOG

NAME:_________________________   GOALS:_________________________

EXERCISES	SETS	REPS	WT	REST	TIME	1 RM	NOTES

DATE:__________   WEIGHT:__________   SLEEP:__________   CALORIES:__________

EXERCISES	SETS	REPS	WT	REST	TIME	1 RM	NOTES

DATE:__________   WEIGHT:__________   SLEEP:__________   CALORIES:__________

EXERCISES	SETS	REPS	WT	REST	TIME	1 RM	NOTES

DATE:__________   WEIGHT:__________   SLEEP:__________   CALORIES:__________

EXERCISES	SETS	REPS	WT	REST	TIME	1 RM	NOTES

DATE:__________   WEIGHT:__________   SLEEP:__________   CALORIES:__________

EXERCISES	SETS	REPS	WT	REST	TIME	1 RM	NOTES

DATE:__________   WEIGHT:__________   SLEEP:__________   CALORIES:__________

WORKOUT LOG

NAME:_________________________   GOALS:_____________________

EXERCISES	SETS	REPS	WT	REST	TIME	1RM	NOTES

DATE:_________   WEIGHT:_________   SLEEP:_________   CALORIES:_________

EXERCISES	SETS	REPS	WT	REST	TIME	1RM	NOTES

DATE:_________   WEIGHT:_________   SLEEP:_________   CALORIES:_________

EXERCISES	SETS	REPS	WT	REST	TIME	1RM	NOTES

DATE:_________   WEIGHT:_________   SLEEP:_________   CALORIES:_________

EXERCISES	SETS	REPS	WT	REST	TIME	1RM	NOTES

DATE:_________   WEIGHT:_________   SLEEP:_________   CALORIES:_________

EXERCISES	SETS	REPS	WT	REST	TIME	1RM	NOTES

DATE:_________   WEIGHT:_________   SLEEP:_________   CALORIES:_________

WORKOUT LOG

NAME:________________________   GOALS:__________________________

EXERCISES	SETS	REPS	WT	REST	TIME	1 RM	NOTES

DATE:__________   WEIGHT:__________   SLEEP:__________   CALORIES:__________

EXERCISES	SETS	REPS	WT	REST	TIME	1 RM	NOTES

DATE:__________   WEIGHT:__________   SLEEP:__________   CALORIES:__________

EXERCISES	SETS	REPS	WT	REST	TIME	1 RM	NOTES

DATE:__________   WEIGHT:__________   SLEEP:__________   CALORIES:__________

EXERCISES	SETS	REPS	WT	REST	TIME	1 RM	NOTES

DATE:__________   WEIGHT:__________   SLEEP:__________   CALORIES:__________

EXERCISES	SETS	REPS	WT	REST	TIME	1 RM	NOTES

DATE:__________   WEIGHT:__________   SLEEP:__________   CALORIES:__________

WORKOUT LOG

NAME:_______________________ GOALS:_______________________

EXERCISES	SETS	REPS	WT	REST	TIME	1 RM	NOTES

DATE:_________ WEIGHT:_________ SLEEP:_________ CALORIES:_________

EXERCISES	SETS	REPS	WT	REST	TIME	1 RM	NOTES

DATE:_________ WEIGHT:_________ SLEEP:_________ CALORIES:_________

EXERCISES	SETS	REPS	WT	REST	TIME	1 RM	NOTES

DATE:_________ WEIGHT:_________ SLEEP:_________ CALORIES:_________

EXERCISES	SETS	REPS	WT	REST	TIME	1 RM	NOTES

DATE:_________ WEIGHT:_________ SLEEP:_________ CALORIES:_________

EXERCISES	SETS	REPS	WT	REST	TIME	1 RM	NOTES

DATE:_________ WEIGHT:_________ SLEEP:_________ CALORIES:_________

WORKOUT LOG

NAME:______________________ GOALS:______________________

EXERCISES	SETS	REPS	WT	REST	TIME	1 RM	NOTES

DATE:__________ WEIGHT:__________ SLEEP:__________ CALORIES:__________

EXERCISES	SETS	REPS	WT	REST	TIME	1 RM	NOTES

DATE:__________ WEIGHT:__________ SLEEP:__________ CALORIES:__________

EXERCISES	SETS	REPS	WT	REST	TIME	1 RM	NOTES

DATE:__________ WEIGHT:__________ SLEEP:__________ CALORIES:__________

EXERCISES	SETS	REPS	WT	REST	TIME	1 RM	NOTES

DATE:__________ WEIGHT:__________ SLEEP:__________ CALORIES:__________

EXERCISES	SETS	REPS	WT	REST	TIME	1 RM	NOTES

DATE:__________ WEIGHT:__________ SLEEP:__________ CALORIES:__________

WORKOUT LOG

NAME:__________________________   GOALS:__________________________

EXERCISES	SETS	REPS	WT	REST	TIME	1 RM	NOTES

DATE:__________   WEIGHT:__________   SLEEP:__________   CALORIES:__________

EXERCISES	SETS	REPS	WT	REST	TIME	1 RM	NOTES

DATE:__________   WEIGHT:__________   SLEEP:__________   CALORIES:__________

EXERCISES	SETS	REPS	WT	REST	TIME	1 RM	NOTES

DATE:__________   WEIGHT:__________   SLEEP:__________   CALORIES:__________

EXERCISES	SETS	REPS	WT	REST	TIME	1 RM	NOTES

DATE:__________   WEIGHT:__________   SLEEP:__________   CALORIES:__________

EXERCISES	SETS	REPS	WT	REST	TIME	1 RM	NOTES

DATE:__________   WEIGHT:__________   SLEEP:__________   CALORIES:__________

WORKOUT LOG

NAME:_______________________   GOALS:_______________________

EXERCISES	SETS	REPS	WT	REST	TIME	1 RM	NOTES

DATE:__________   WEIGHT:__________   SLEEP:__________   CALORIES:__________

EXERCISES	SETS	REPS	WT	REST	TIME	1 RM	NOTES

DATE:__________   WEIGHT:__________   SLEEP:__________   CALORIES:__________

EXERCISES	SETS	REPS	WT	REST	TIME	1 RM	NOTES

DATE:__________   WEIGHT:__________   SLEEP:__________   CALORIES:__________

EXERCISES	SETS	REPS	WT	REST	TIME	1 RM	NOTES

DATE:__________   WEIGHT:__________   SLEEP:__________   CALORIES:__________

EXERCISES	SETS	REPS	WT	REST	TIME	1 RM	NOTES

DATE:__________   WEIGHT:__________   SLEEP:__________   CALORIES:__________

WORKOUT LOG

NAME:________________________   GOALS:________________________

EXERCISES	SETS	REPS	WT	REST	TIME	1 RM	NOTES

DATE:__________   WEIGHT:__________   SLEEP:__________   CALORIES:__________

EXERCISES	SETS	REPS	WT	REST	TIME	1 RM	NOTES

DATE:__________   WEIGHT:__________   SLEEP:__________   CALORIES:__________

EXERCISES	SETS	REPS	WT	REST	TIME	1 RM	NOTES

DATE:__________   WEIGHT:__________   SLEEP:__________   CALORIES:__________

EXERCISES	SETS	REPS	WT	REST	TIME	1 RM	NOTES

DATE:__________   WEIGHT:__________   SLEEP:__________   CALORIES:__________

EXERCISES	SETS	REPS	WT	REST	TIME	1 RM	NOTES

DATE:__________   WEIGHT:__________   SLEEP:__________   CALORIES:__________

WORKOUT LOG

NAME:________________________   GOALS:__________________________

EXERCISES	SETS	REPS	WT	REST	TIME	1 RM	NOTES

DATE:__________   WEIGHT:__________   SLEEP:__________   CALORIES:__________

EXERCISES	SETS	REPS	WT	REST	TIME	1 RM	NOTES

DATE:__________   WEIGHT:__________   SLEEP:__________   CALORIES:__________

EXERCISES	SETS	REPS	WT	REST	TIME	1 RM	NOTES

DATE:__________   WEIGHT:__________   SLEEP:__________   CALORIES:__________

EXERCISES	SETS	REPS	WT	REST	TIME	1 RM	NOTES

DATE:__________   WEIGHT:__________   SLEEP:__________   CALORIES:__________

EXERCISES	SETS	REPS	WT	REST	TIME	1 RM	NOTES

DATE:__________   WEIGHT:__________   SLEEP:__________   CALORIES:__________

WORKOUT LOG

NAME:_________________________ GOALS:_____________________

EXERCISES	SETS	REPS	WT	REST	TIME	1 RM	NOTES

DATE:_________ WEIGHT:_________ SLEEP:_________ CALORIES:_________

EXERCISES	SETS	REPS	WT	REST	TIME	1 RM	NOTES

DATE:_________ WEIGHT:_________ SLEEP:_________ CALORIES:_________

EXERCISES	SETS	REPS	WT	REST	TIME	1 RM	NOTES

DATE:_________ WEIGHT:_________ SLEEP:_________ CALORIES:_________

EXERCISES	SETS	REPS	WT	REST	TIME	1 RM	NOTES

DATE:_________ WEIGHT:_________ SLEEP:_________ CALORIES:_________

EXERCISES	SETS	REPS	WT	REST	TIME	1 RM	NOTES

DATE:_________ WEIGHT:_________ SLEEP:_________ CALORIES:_________

WORKOUT LOG

NAME:______________________   GOALS:______________________

EXERCISES	SETS	REPS	WT	REST	TIME	1 RM	NOTES

DATE:__________   WEIGHT:__________   SLEEP:__________   CALORIES:__________

EXERCISES	SETS	REPS	WT	REST	TIME	1 RM	NOTES

DATE:__________   WEIGHT:__________   SLEEP:__________   CALORIES:__________

EXERCISES	SETS	REPS	WT	REST	TIME	1 RM	NOTES

DATE:__________   WEIGHT:__________   SLEEP:__________   CALORIES:__________

EXERCISES	SETS	REPS	WT	REST	TIME	1 RM	NOTES

DATE:__________   WEIGHT:__________   SLEEP:__________   CALORIES:__________

EXERCISES	SETS	REPS	WT	REST	TIME	1 RM	NOTES

DATE:__________   WEIGHT:__________   SLEEP:__________   CALORIES:__________

WORKOUT LOG

NAME:_________________________ GOALS:___________________________

EXERCISES	SETS	REPS	WT	REST	TIME	1RM	NOTES

DATE:__________ WEIGHT:__________ SLEEP:__________ CALORIES:__________

EXERCISES	SETS	REPS	WT	REST	TIME	1RM	NOTES

DATE:__________ WEIGHT:__________ SLEEP:__________ CALORIES:__________

EXERCISES	SETS	REPS	WT	REST	TIME	1RM	NOTES

DATE:__________ WEIGHT:__________ SLEEP:__________ CALORIES:__________

EXERCISES	SETS	REPS	WT	REST	TIME	1RM	NOTES

DATE:__________ WEIGHT:__________ SLEEP:__________ CALORIES:__________

EXERCISES	SETS	REPS	WT	REST	TIME	1RM	NOTES

DATE:__________ WEIGHT:__________ SLEEP:__________ CALORIES:__________

WORKOUT LOG

NAME:________________________   GOALS:________________________

EXERCISES	SETS	REPS	WT	REST	TIME	1 RM	NOTES

DATE:__________   WEIGHT:__________   SLEEP:__________   CALORIES:__________

EXERCISES	SETS	REPS	WT	REST	TIME	1 RM	NOTES

DATE:__________   WEIGHT:__________   SLEEP:__________   CALORIES:__________

EXERCISES	SETS	REPS	WT	REST	TIME	1 RM	NOTES

DATE:__________   WEIGHT:__________   SLEEP:__________   CALORIES:__________

EXERCISES	SETS	REPS	WT	REST	TIME	1 RM	NOTES

DATE:__________   WEIGHT:__________   SLEEP:__________   CALORIES:__________

EXERCISES	SETS	REPS	WT	REST	TIME	1 RM	NOTES

DATE:__________   WEIGHT:__________   SLEEP:__________   CALORIES:__________

WORKOUT LOG

NAME:____________________ GOALS:____________________

EXERCISES	SETS	REPS	WT	REST	TIME	1 RM	NOTES

DATE:__________ WEIGHT:__________ SLEEP:__________ CALORIES:__________

EXERCISES	SETS	REPS	WT	REST	TIME	1 RM	NOTES

DATE:__________ WEIGHT:__________ SLEEP:__________ CALORIES:__________

EXERCISES	SETS	REPS	WT	REST	TIME	1 RM	NOTES

DATE:__________ WEIGHT:__________ SLEEP:__________ CALORIES:__________

EXERCISES	SETS	REPS	WT	REST	TIME	1 RM	NOTES

DATE:__________ WEIGHT:__________ SLEEP:__________ CALORIES:__________

EXERCISES	SETS	REPS	WT	REST	TIME	1 RM	NOTES

DATE:__________ WEIGHT:__________ SLEEP:__________ CALORIES:__________

WORKOUT LOG

NAME: _________________________   GOALS: _________________________

EXERCISES	SETS	REPS	WT	REST	TIME	1 RM	NOTES

DATE: __________   WEIGHT: __________   SLEEP: __________   CALORIES: __________

EXERCISES	SETS	REPS	WT	REST	TIME	1 RM	NOTES

DATE: __________   WEIGHT: __________   SLEEP: __________   CALORIES: __________

EXERCISES	SETS	REPS	WT	REST	TIME	1 RM	NOTES

DATE: __________   WEIGHT: __________   SLEEP: __________   CALORIES: __________

EXERCISES	SETS	REPS	WT	REST	TIME	1 RM	NOTES

DATE: __________   WEIGHT: __________   SLEEP: __________   CALORIES: __________

EXERCISES	SETS	REPS	WT	REST	TIME	1 RM	NOTES

DATE: __________   WEIGHT: __________   SLEEP: __________   CALORIES: __________

WORKOUT LOG

NAME:_________________________   GOALS:_________________________

EXERCISES	SETS	REPS	WT	REST	TIME	1 RM	NOTES

DATE:__________   WEIGHT:__________   SLEEP:__________   CALORIES:__________

EXERCISES	SETS	REPS	WT	REST	TIME	1 RM	NOTES

DATE:__________   WEIGHT:__________   SLEEP:__________   CALORIES:__________

EXERCISES	SETS	REPS	WT	REST	TIME	1 RM	NOTES

DATE:__________   WEIGHT:__________   SLEEP:__________   CALORIES:__________

EXERCISES	SETS	REPS	WT	REST	TIME	1 RM	NOTES

DATE:__________   WEIGHT:__________   SLEEP:__________   CALORIES:__________

EXERCISES	SETS	REPS	WT	REST	TIME	1 RM	NOTES

DATE:__________   WEIGHT:__________   SLEEP:__________   CALORIES:__________

WORKOUT LOG

NAME:_________________________ GOALS:___________________________

EXERCISES	SETS	REPS	WT	REST	TIME	1 RM	NOTES

DATE:__________ WEIGHT:__________ SLEEP:__________ CALORIES:__________

EXERCISES	SETS	REPS	WT	REST	TIME	1 RM	NOTES

DATE:__________ WEIGHT:__________ SLEEP:__________ CALORIES:__________

EXERCISES	SETS	REPS	WT	REST	TIME	1 RM	NOTES

DATE:__________ WEIGHT:__________ SLEEP:__________ CALORIES:__________

EXERCISES	SETS	REPS	WT	REST	TIME	1 RM	NOTES

DATE:__________ WEIGHT:__________ SLEEP:__________ CALORIES:__________

EXERCISES	SETS	REPS	WT	REST	TIME	1 RM	NOTES

DATE:__________ WEIGHT:__________ SLEEP:__________ CALORIES:__________

WORKOUT LOG

NAME:___________________________ GOALS:___________________________

EXERCISES	SETS	REPS	WT	REST	TIME	1 RM	NOTES

DATE:__________ WEIGHT:__________ SLEEP:__________ CALORIES:__________

EXERCISES	SETS	REPS	WT	REST	TIME	1 RM	NOTES

DATE:__________ WEIGHT:__________ SLEEP:__________ CALORIES:__________

EXERCISES	SETS	REPS	WT	REST	TIME	1 RM	NOTES

DATE:__________ WEIGHT:__________ SLEEP:__________ CALORIES:__________

EXERCISES	SETS	REPS	WT	REST	TIME	1 RM	NOTES

DATE:__________ WEIGHT:__________ SLEEP:__________ CALORIES:__________

EXERCISES	SETS	REPS	WT	REST	TIME	1 RM	NOTES

DATE:__________ WEIGHT:__________ SLEEP:__________ CALORIES:__________

WORKOUT LOG

NAME:____________________________   GOALS:____________________________

EXERCISES	SETS	REPS	WT	REST	TIME	1 RM	NOTES

DATE:__________   WEIGHT:__________   SLEEP:__________   CALORIES:__________

EXERCISES	SETS	REPS	WT	REST	TIME	1 RM	NOTES

DATE:__________   WEIGHT:__________   SLEEP:__________   CALORIES:__________

EXERCISES	SETS	REPS	WT	REST	TIME	1 RM	NOTES

DATE:__________   WEIGHT:__________   SLEEP:__________   CALORIES:__________

EXERCISES	SETS	REPS	WT	REST	TIME	1 RM	NOTES

DATE:__________   WEIGHT:__________   SLEEP:__________   CALORIES:__________

EXERCISES	SETS	REPS	WT	REST	TIME	1 RM	NOTES

DATE:__________   WEIGHT:__________   SLEEP:__________   CALORIES:__________

WORKOUT LOG

NAME:_______________________   GOALS:____________________

EXERCISES	SETS	REPS	WT	REST	TIME	1 RM	NOTES

DATE:_________   WEIGHT:_________   SLEEP:_________   CALORIES:_________

EXERCISES	SETS	REPS	WT	REST	TIME	1 RM	NOTES

DATE:_________   WEIGHT:_________   SLEEP:_________   CALORIES:_________

EXERCISES	SETS	REPS	WT	REST	TIME	1 RM	NOTES

DATE:_________   WEIGHT:_________   SLEEP:_________   CALORIES:_________

EXERCISES	SETS	REPS	WT	REST	TIME	1 RM	NOTES

DATE:_________   WEIGHT:_________   SLEEP:_________   CALORIES:_________

EXERCISES	SETS	REPS	WT	REST	TIME	1 RM	NOTES

DATE:_________   WEIGHT:_________   SLEEP:_________   CALORIES:_________

WORKOUT LOG

NAME:_________________________ GOALS:_________________________

EXERCISES	SETS	REPS	WT	REST	TIME	1 RM	NOTES

DATE:_________ WEIGHT:_________ SLEEP:_________ CALORIES:_________

EXERCISES	SETS	REPS	WT	REST	TIME	1 RM	NOTES

DATE:_________ WEIGHT:_________ SLEEP:_________ CALORIES:_________

EXERCISES	SETS	REPS	WT	REST	TIME	1 RM	NOTES

DATE:_________ WEIGHT:_________ SLEEP:_________ CALORIES:_________

EXERCISES	SETS	REPS	WT	REST	TIME	1 RM	NOTES

DATE:_________ WEIGHT:_________ SLEEP:_________ CALORIES:_________

EXERCISES	SETS	REPS	WT	REST	TIME	1 RM	NOTES

DATE:_________ WEIGHT:_________ SLEEP:_________ CALORIES:_________

WORKOUT LOG

NAME:_________________________ GOALS:_________________________

EXERCISES	SETS	REPS	WT	REST	TIME	1 RM	NOTES

DATE:__________ WEIGHT:__________ SLEEP:__________ CALORIES:__________

EXERCISES	SETS	REPS	WT	REST	TIME	1 RM	NOTES

DATE:__________ WEIGHT:__________ SLEEP:__________ CALORIES:__________

EXERCISES	SETS	REPS	WT	REST	TIME	1 RM	NOTES

DATE:__________ WEIGHT:__________ SLEEP:__________ CALORIES:__________

EXERCISES	SETS	REPS	WT	REST	TIME	1 RM	NOTES

DATE:__________ WEIGHT:__________ SLEEP:__________ CALORIES:__________

EXERCISES	SETS	REPS	WT	REST	TIME	1 RM	NOTES

DATE:__________ WEIGHT:__________ SLEEP:__________ CALORIES:__________

WORKOUT LOG

NAME:_________________________   GOALS:_________________________

EXERCISES	SETS	REPS	WT	REST	TIME	1 RM	NOTES

DATE:__________   WEIGHT:__________   SLEEP:__________   CALORIES:__________

EXERCISES	SETS	REPS	WT	REST	TIME	1 RM	NOTES

DATE:__________   WEIGHT:__________   SLEEP:__________   CALORIES:__________

EXERCISES	SETS	REPS	WT	REST	TIME	1 RM	NOTES

DATE:__________   WEIGHT:__________   SLEEP:__________   CALORIES:__________

EXERCISES	SETS	REPS	WT	REST	TIME	1 RM	NOTES

DATE:__________   WEIGHT:__________   SLEEP:__________   CALORIES:__________

EXERCISES	SETS	REPS	WT	REST	TIME	1 RM	NOTES

DATE:__________   WEIGHT:__________   SLEEP:__________   CALORIES:__________

WORKOUT LOG

NAME:_______________________   GOALS:_______________________

EXERCISES	SETS	REPS	WT	REST	TIME	1 RM	NOTES

DATE:__________   WEIGHT:__________   SLEEP:__________   CALORIES:__________

EXERCISES	SETS	REPS	WT	REST	TIME	1 RM	NOTES

DATE:__________   WEIGHT:__________   SLEEP:__________   CALORIES:__________

EXERCISES	SETS	REPS	WT	REST	TIME	1 RM	NOTES

DATE:__________   WEIGHT:__________   SLEEP:__________   CALORIES:__________

EXERCISES	SETS	REPS	WT	REST	TIME	1 RM	NOTES

DATE:__________   WEIGHT:__________   SLEEP:__________   CALORIES:__________

EXERCISES	SETS	REPS	WT	REST	TIME	1 RM	NOTES

DATE:__________   WEIGHT:__________   SLEEP:__________   CALORIES:__________

WORKOUT LOG

NAME:________________________   GOALS:________________________

EXERCISES	SETS	REPS	WT	REST	TIME	1 RM	NOTES

DATE:__________   WEIGHT:__________   SLEEP:__________   CALORIES:__________

EXERCISES	SETS	REPS	WT	REST	TIME	1 RM	NOTES

DATE:__________   WEIGHT:__________   SLEEP:__________   CALORIES:__________

EXERCISES	SETS	REPS	WT	REST	TIME	1 RM	NOTES

DATE:__________   WEIGHT:__________   SLEEP:__________   CALORIES:__________

EXERCISES	SETS	REPS	WT	REST	TIME	1 RM	NOTES

DATE:__________   WEIGHT:__________   SLEEP:__________   CALORIES:__________

EXERCISES	SETS	REPS	WT	REST	TIME	1 RM	NOTES

DATE:__________   WEIGHT:__________   SLEEP:__________   CALORIES:__________

WORKOUT LOG

NAME:____________________________   GOALS:____________________________

EXERCISES	SETS	REPS	WT	REST	TIME	1 RM	NOTES

DATE:__________   WEIGHT:__________   SLEEP:__________   CALORIES:__________

EXERCISES	SETS	REPS	WT	REST	TIME	1 RM	NOTES

DATE:__________   WEIGHT:__________   SLEEP:__________   CALORIES:__________

EXERCISES	SETS	REPS	WT	REST	TIME	1 RM	NOTES

DATE:__________   WEIGHT:__________   SLEEP:__________   CALORIES:__________

EXERCISES	SETS	REPS	WT	REST	TIME	1 RM	NOTES

DATE:__________   WEIGHT:__________   SLEEP:__________   CALORIES:__________

EXERCISES	SETS	REPS	WT	REST	TIME	1 RM	NOTES

DATE:__________   WEIGHT:__________   SLEEP:__________   CALORIES:__________

WORKOUT LOG

NAME:________________________   GOALS:________________________

EXERCISES	SETS	REPS	WT	REST	TIME	1 RM	NOTES

DATE:__________   WEIGHT:__________   SLEEP:__________   CALORIES:__________

EXERCISES	SETS	REPS	WT	REST	TIME	1 RM	NOTES

DATE:__________   WEIGHT:__________   SLEEP:__________   CALORIES:__________

EXERCISES	SETS	REPS	WT	REST	TIME	1 RM	NOTES

DATE:__________   WEIGHT:__________   SLEEP:__________   CALORIES:__________

EXERCISES	SETS	REPS	WT	REST	TIME	1 RM	NOTES

DATE:__________   WEIGHT:__________   SLEEP:__________   CALORIES:__________

EXERCISES	SETS	REPS	WT	REST	TIME	1 RM	NOTES

DATE:__________   WEIGHT:__________   SLEEP:__________   CALORIES:__________

WORKOUT LOG

NAME:_________________________ GOALS:_____________________

EXERCISES	SETS	REPS	WT	REST	TIME	1 RM	NOTES

DATE:__________ WEIGHT:__________ SLEEP:__________ CALORIES:__________

EXERCISES	SETS	REPS	WT	REST	TIME	1 RM	NOTES

DATE:__________ WEIGHT:__________ SLEEP:__________ CALORIES:__________

EXERCISES	SETS	REPS	WT	REST	TIME	1 RM	NOTES

DATE:__________ WEIGHT:__________ SLEEP:__________ CALORIES:__________

EXERCISES	SETS	REPS	WT	REST	TIME	1 RM	NOTES

DATE:__________ WEIGHT:__________ SLEEP:__________ CALORIES:__________

EXERCISES	SETS	REPS	WT	REST	TIME	1 RM	NOTES

DATE:__________ WEIGHT:__________ SLEEP:__________ CALORIES:__________

WORKOUT LOG

NAME:_________________________   GOALS:_________________________

EXERCISES	SETS	REPS	WT	REST	TIME	1 RM	NOTES

DATE:_________   WEIGHT:_________   SLEEP:_________   CALORIES:_________

EXERCISES	SETS	REPS	WT	REST	TIME	1 RM	NOTES

DATE:_________   WEIGHT:_________   SLEEP:_________   CALORIES:_________

EXERCISES	SETS	REPS	WT	REST	TIME	1 RM	NOTES

DATE:_________   WEIGHT:_________   SLEEP:_________   CALORIES:_________

EXERCISES	SETS	REPS	WT	REST	TIME	1 RM	NOTES

DATE:_________   WEIGHT:_________   SLEEP:_________   CALORIES:_________

EXERCISES	SETS	REPS	WT	REST	TIME	1 RM	NOTES

DATE:_________   WEIGHT:_________   SLEEP:_________   CALORIES:_________

WORKOUT LOG

NAME:_________________________   GOALS:___________________________

EXERCISES	SETS	REPS	WT	REST	TIME	1 RM	NOTES

DATE:__________   WEIGHT:__________   SLEEP:__________   CALORIES:__________

EXERCISES	SETS	REPS	WT	REST	TIME	1 RM	NOTES

DATE:__________   WEIGHT:__________   SLEEP:__________   CALORIES:__________

EXERCISES	SETS	REPS	WT	REST	TIME	1 RM	NOTES

DATE:__________   WEIGHT:__________   SLEEP:__________   CALORIES:__________

EXERCISES	SETS	REPS	WT	REST	TIME	1 RM	NOTES

DATE:__________   WEIGHT:__________   SLEEP:__________   CALORIES:__________

EXERCISES	SETS	REPS	WT	REST	TIME	1 RM	NOTES

DATE:__________   WEIGHT:__________   SLEEP:__________   CALORIES:__________

WORKOUT LOG

NAME:_________________________   GOALS:_____________________________

EXERCISES	SETS	REPS	WT	REST	TIME	1 RM	NOTES

DATE:__________   WEIGHT:__________   SLEEP:__________   CALORIES:__________

EXERCISES	SETS	REPS	WT	REST	TIME	1 RM	NOTES

DATE:__________   WEIGHT:__________   SLEEP:__________   CALORIES:__________

EXERCISES	SETS	REPS	WT	REST	TIME	1 RM	NOTES

DATE:__________   WEIGHT:__________   SLEEP:__________   CALORIES:__________

EXERCISES	SETS	REPS	WT	REST	TIME	1 RM	NOTES

DATE:__________   WEIGHT:__________   SLEEP:__________   CALORIES:__________

EXERCISES	SETS	REPS	WT	REST	TIME	1 RM	NOTES

DATE:__________   WEIGHT:__________   SLEEP:__________   CALORIES:__________

WORKOUT LOG

NAME:_______________________   GOALS:_______________________

EXERCISES	SETS	REPS	WT	REST	TIME	1 RM	NOTES

DATE:__________   WEIGHT:__________   SLEEP:__________   CALORIES:__________

EXERCISES	SETS	REPS	WT	REST	TIME	1 RM	NOTES

DATE:__________   WEIGHT:__________   SLEEP:__________   CALORIES:__________

EXERCISES	SETS	REPS	WT	REST	TIME	1 RM	NOTES

DATE:__________   WEIGHT:__________   SLEEP:__________   CALORIES:__________

EXERCISES	SETS	REPS	WT	REST	TIME	1 RM	NOTES

DATE:__________   WEIGHT:__________   SLEEP:__________   CALORIES:__________

EXERCISES	SETS	REPS	WT	REST	TIME	1 RM	NOTES

DATE:__________   WEIGHT:__________   SLEEP:__________   CALORIES:__________

WORKOUT LOG

NAME:___________________________   GOALS:___________________________

EXERCISES	SETS	REPS	WT	REST	TIME	1 RM	NOTES

DATE:___________   WEIGHT:___________   SLEEP:___________   CALORIES:___________

EXERCISES	SETS	REPS	WT	REST	TIME	1 RM	NOTES

DATE:___________   WEIGHT:___________   SLEEP:___________   CALORIES:___________

EXERCISES	SETS	REPS	WT	REST	TIME	1 RM	NOTES

DATE:___________   WEIGHT:___________   SLEEP:___________   CALORIES:___________

EXERCISES	SETS	REPS	WT	REST	TIME	1 RM	NOTES

DATE:___________   WEIGHT:___________   SLEEP:___________   CALORIES:___________

EXERCISES	SETS	REPS	WT	REST	TIME	1 RM	NOTES

DATE:___________   WEIGHT:___________   SLEEP:___________   CALORIES:___________

WORKOUT LOG

NAME:__________________________ GOALS:__________________________

EXERCISES	SETS	REPS	WT	REST	TIME	1 RM	NOTES

DATE:__________ WEIGHT:__________ SLEEP:__________ CALORIES:__________

EXERCISES	SETS	REPS	WT	REST	TIME	1 RM	NOTES

DATE:__________ WEIGHT:__________ SLEEP:__________ CALORIES:__________

EXERCISES	SETS	REPS	WT	REST	TIME	1 RM	NOTES

DATE:__________ WEIGHT:__________ SLEEP:__________ CALORIES:__________

EXERCISES	SETS	REPS	WT	REST	TIME	1 RM	NOTES

DATE:__________ WEIGHT:__________ SLEEP:__________ CALORIES:__________

EXERCISES	SETS	REPS	WT	REST	TIME	1 RM	NOTES

DATE:__________ WEIGHT:__________ SLEEP:__________ CALORIES:__________

WORKOUT LOG

NAME:______________________   GOALS:______________________

EXERCISES	SETS	REPS	WT	REST	TIME	1 RM	NOTES

DATE:__________   WEIGHT:__________   SLEEP:__________   CALORIES:__________

EXERCISES	SETS	REPS	WT	REST	TIME	1 RM	NOTES

DATE:__________   WEIGHT:__________   SLEEP:__________   CALORIES:__________

EXERCISES	SETS	REPS	WT	REST	TIME	1 RM	NOTES

DATE:__________   WEIGHT:__________   SLEEP:__________   CALORIES:__________

EXERCISES	SETS	REPS	WT	REST	TIME	1 RM	NOTES

DATE:__________   WEIGHT:__________   SLEEP:__________   CALORIES:__________

EXERCISES	SETS	REPS	WT	REST	TIME	1 RM	NOTES

DATE:__________   WEIGHT:__________   SLEEP:__________   CALORIES:__________

WORKOUT LOG

NAME:___________________________   GOALS:___________________________

EXERCISES	SETS	REPS	WT	REST	TIME	1 RM	NOTES

DATE:__________   WEIGHT:__________   SLEEP:__________   CALORIES:__________

EXERCISES	SETS	REPS	WT	REST	TIME	1 RM	NOTES

DATE:__________   WEIGHT:__________   SLEEP:__________   CALORIES:__________

EXERCISES	SETS	REPS	WT	REST	TIME	1 RM	NOTES

DATE:__________   WEIGHT:__________   SLEEP:__________   CALORIES:__________

EXERCISES	SETS	REPS	WT	REST	TIME	1 RM	NOTES

DATE:__________   WEIGHT:__________   SLEEP:__________   CALORIES:__________

EXERCISES	SETS	REPS	WT	REST	TIME	1 RM	NOTES

DATE:__________   WEIGHT:__________   SLEEP:__________   CALORIES:__________

WORKOUT LOG

NAME:______________________ GOALS:______________________

EXERCISES	SETS	REPS	WT	REST	TIME	1 RM	NOTES

DATE:__________ WEIGHT:__________ SLEEP:__________ CALORIES:__________

EXERCISES	SETS	REPS	WT	REST	TIME	1 RM	NOTES

DATE:__________ WEIGHT:__________ SLEEP:__________ CALORIES:__________

EXERCISES	SETS	REPS	WT	REST	TIME	1 RM	NOTES

DATE:__________ WEIGHT:__________ SLEEP:__________ CALORIES:__________

EXERCISES	SETS	REPS	WT	REST	TIME	1 RM	NOTES

DATE:__________ WEIGHT:__________ SLEEP:__________ CALORIES:__________

EXERCISES	SETS	REPS	WT	REST	TIME	1 RM	NOTES

DATE:__________ WEIGHT:__________ SLEEP:__________ CALORIES:__________

WORKOUT LOG

NAME:_________________________ **GOALS:**_____________________

EXERCISES	SETS	REPS	WT	REST	TIME	1 RM	NOTES

DATE:__________ **WEIGHT:**__________ **SLEEP:**__________ **CALORIES:**__________

EXERCISES	SETS	REPS	WT	REST	TIME	1 RM	NOTES

DATE:__________ **WEIGHT:**__________ **SLEEP:**__________ **CALORIES:**__________

EXERCISES	SETS	REPS	WT	REST	TIME	1 RM	NOTES

DATE:__________ **WEIGHT:**__________ **SLEEP:**__________ **CALORIES:**__________

EXERCISES	SETS	REPS	WT	REST	TIME	1 RM	NOTES

DATE:__________ **WEIGHT:**__________ **SLEEP:**__________ **CALORIES:**__________

EXERCISES	SETS	REPS	WT	REST	TIME	1 RM	NOTES

DATE:__________ **WEIGHT:**__________ **SLEEP:**__________ **CALORIES:**__________

WORKOUT LOG

NAME:_________________________ GOALS:_________________________

EXERCISES	SETS	REPS	WT	REST	TIME	1 RM	NOTES

DATE:_________ WEIGHT:_________ SLEEP:_________ CALORIES:_________

EXERCISES	SETS	REPS	WT	REST	TIME	1 RM	NOTES

DATE:_________ WEIGHT:_________ SLEEP:_________ CALORIES:_________

EXERCISES	SETS	REPS	WT	REST	TIME	1 RM	NOTES

DATE:_________ WEIGHT:_________ SLEEP:_________ CALORIES:_________

EXERCISES	SETS	REPS	WT	REST	TIME	1 RM	NOTES

DATE:_________ WEIGHT:_________ SLEEP:_________ CALORIES:_________

EXERCISES	SETS	REPS	WT	REST	TIME	1 RM	NOTES

DATE:_________ WEIGHT:_________ SLEEP:_________ CALORIES:_________

WORKOUT LOG

NAME:_________________________   GOALS:_________________________

EXERCISES	SETS	REPS	WT	REST	TIME	1 RM	NOTES

DATE:_________   WEIGHT:_________   SLEEP:_________   CALORIES:_________

EXERCISES	SETS	REPS	WT	REST	TIME	1 RM	NOTES

DATE:_________   WEIGHT:_________   SLEEP:_________   CALORIES:_________

EXERCISES	SETS	REPS	WT	REST	TIME	1 RM	NOTES

DATE:_________   WEIGHT:_________   SLEEP:_________   CALORIES:_________

EXERCISES	SETS	REPS	WT	REST	TIME	1 RM	NOTES

DATE:_________   WEIGHT:_________   SLEEP:_________   CALORIES:_________

EXERCISES	SETS	REPS	WT	REST	TIME	1 RM	NOTES

DATE:_________   WEIGHT:_________   SLEEP:_________   CALORIES:_________

WORKOUT LOG

NAME:_________________________ GOALS:_________________________

EXERCISES	SETS	REPS	WT	REST	TIME	1 RM	NOTES

DATE:__________ WEIGHT:__________ SLEEP:__________ CALORIES:__________

EXERCISES	SETS	REPS	WT	REST	TIME	1 RM	NOTES

DATE:__________ WEIGHT:__________ SLEEP:__________ CALORIES:__________

EXERCISES	SETS	REPS	WT	REST	TIME	1 RM	NOTES

DATE:__________ WEIGHT:__________ SLEEP:__________ CALORIES:__________

EXERCISES	SETS	REPS	WT	REST	TIME	1 RM	NOTES

DATE:__________ WEIGHT:__________ SLEEP:__________ CALORIES:__________

EXERCISES	SETS	REPS	WT	REST	TIME	1 RM	NOTES

DATE:__________ WEIGHT:__________ SLEEP:__________ CALORIES:__________

WORKOUT LOG

NAME:__________________________   GOALS:__________________________

EXERCISES	SETS	REPS	WT	REST	TIME	1 RM	NOTES

DATE:__________   WEIGHT:__________   SLEEP:__________   CALORIES:__________

EXERCISES	SETS	REPS	WT	REST	TIME	1 RM	NOTES

DATE:__________   WEIGHT:__________   SLEEP:__________   CALORIES:__________

EXERCISES	SETS	REPS	WT	REST	TIME	1 RM	NOTES

DATE:__________   WEIGHT:__________   SLEEP:__________   CALORIES:__________

EXERCISES	SETS	REPS	WT	REST	TIME	1 RM	NOTES

DATE:__________   WEIGHT:__________   SLEEP:__________   CALORIES:__________

EXERCISES	SETS	REPS	WT	REST	TIME	1 RM	NOTES

DATE:__________   WEIGHT:__________   SLEEP:__________   CALORIES:__________

WORKOUT LOG

NAME:________________________ GOALS:________________________

EXERCISES	SETS	REPS	WT	REST	TIME	1 RM	NOTES

DATE:__________   WEIGHT:__________   SLEEP:__________   CALORIES:__________

EXERCISES	SETS	REPS	WT	REST	TIME	1 RM	NOTES

DATE:__________   WEIGHT:__________   SLEEP:__________   CALORIES:__________

EXERCISES	SETS	REPS	WT	REST	TIME	1 RM	NOTES

DATE:__________   WEIGHT:__________   SLEEP:__________   CALORIES:__________

EXERCISES	SETS	REPS	WT	REST	TIME	1 RM	NOTES

DATE:__________   WEIGHT:__________   SLEEP:__________   CALORIES:__________

EXERCISES	SETS	REPS	WT	REST	TIME	1 RM	NOTES

DATE:__________   WEIGHT:__________   SLEEP:__________   CALORIES:__________

WORKOUT LOG

NAME:________________________   GOALS:__________________________

EXERCISES	SETS	REPS	WT	REST	TIME	1 RM	NOTES

DATE:__________   WEIGHT:__________   SLEEP:__________   CALORIES:__________

EXERCISES	SETS	REPS	WT	REST	TIME	1 RM	NOTES

DATE:__________   WEIGHT:__________   SLEEP:__________   CALORIES:__________

EXERCISES	SETS	REPS	WT	REST	TIME	1 RM	NOTES

DATE:__________   WEIGHT:__________   SLEEP:__________   CALORIES:__________

EXERCISES	SETS	REPS	WT	REST	TIME	1 RM	NOTES

DATE:__________   WEIGHT:__________   SLEEP:__________   CALORIES:__________

EXERCISES	SETS	REPS	WT	REST	TIME	1 RM	NOTES

DATE:__________   WEIGHT:__________   SLEEP:__________   CALORIES:__________

WORKOUT LOG

NAME:________________________ GOALS:________________________

EXERCISES	SETS	REPS	WT	REST	TIME	1 RM	NOTES

DATE:__________ WEIGHT:__________ SLEEP:__________ CALORIES:__________

EXERCISES	SETS	REPS	WT	REST	TIME	1 RM	NOTES

DATE:__________ WEIGHT:__________ SLEEP:__________ CALORIES:__________

EXERCISES	SETS	REPS	WT	REST	TIME	1 RM	NOTES

DATE:__________ WEIGHT:__________ SLEEP:__________ CALORIES:__________

EXERCISES	SETS	REPS	WT	REST	TIME	1 RM	NOTES

DATE:__________ WEIGHT:__________ SLEEP:__________ CALORIES:__________

EXERCISES	SETS	REPS	WT	REST	TIME	1 RM	NOTES

DATE:__________ WEIGHT:__________ SLEEP:__________ CALORIES:__________

WORKOUT LOG

NAME:_______________________   GOALS:_______________________

EXERCISES	SETS	REPS	WT	REST	TIME	1 RM	NOTES

DATE:__________   WEIGHT:__________   SLEEP:__________   CALORIES:__________

EXERCISES	SETS	REPS	WT	REST	TIME	1 RM	NOTES

DATE:__________   WEIGHT:__________   SLEEP:__________   CALORIES:__________

EXERCISES	SETS	REPS	WT	REST	TIME	1 RM	NOTES

DATE:__________   WEIGHT:__________   SLEEP:__________   CALORIES:__________

EXERCISES	SETS	REPS	WT	REST	TIME	1 RM	NOTES

DATE:__________   WEIGHT:__________   SLEEP:__________   CALORIES:__________

EXERCISES	SETS	REPS	WT	REST	TIME	1 RM	NOTES

DATE:__________   WEIGHT:__________   SLEEP:__________   CALORIES:__________

WORKOUT LOG

NAME:________________________   GOALS:____________________

EXERCISES	SETS	REPS	WT	REST	TIME	1 RM	NOTES

DATE:__________   WEIGHT:__________   SLEEP:__________   CALORIES:__________

EXERCISES	SETS	REPS	WT	REST	TIME	1 RM	NOTES

DATE:__________   WEIGHT:__________   SLEEP:__________   CALORIES:__________

EXERCISES	SETS	REPS	WT	REST	TIME	1 RM	NOTES

DATE:__________   WEIGHT:__________   SLEEP:__________   CALORIES:__________

EXERCISES	SETS	REPS	WT	REST	TIME	1 RM	NOTES

DATE:__________   WEIGHT:__________   SLEEP:__________   CALORIES:__________

EXERCISES	SETS	REPS	WT	REST	TIME	1 RM	NOTES

DATE:__________   WEIGHT:__________   SLEEP:__________   CALORIES:__________

WORKOUT LOG

NAME:________________________ GOALS:________________________

EXERCISES	SETS	REPS	WT	REST	TIME	1 RM	NOTES

DATE:__________   WEIGHT:__________   SLEEP:__________   CALORIES:__________

EXERCISES	SETS	REPS	WT	REST	TIME	1 RM	NOTES

DATE:__________   WEIGHT:__________   SLEEP:__________   CALORIES:__________

EXERCISES	SETS	REPS	WT	REST	TIME	1 RM	NOTES

DATE:__________   WEIGHT:__________   SLEEP:__________   CALORIES:__________

EXERCISES	SETS	REPS	WT	REST	TIME	1 RM	NOTES

DATE:__________   WEIGHT:__________   SLEEP:__________   CALORIES:__________

EXERCISES	SETS	REPS	WT	REST	TIME	1 RM	NOTES

DATE:__________   WEIGHT:__________   SLEEP:__________   CALORIES:__________

WORKOUT LOG

NAME:_____________________________   GOALS:_____________________________

EXERCISES	SETS	REPS	WT	REST	TIME	1 RM	NOTES

DATE:__________   WEIGHT:__________   SLEEP:__________   CALORIES:__________

EXERCISES	SETS	REPS	WT	REST	TIME	1 RM	NOTES

DATE:__________   WEIGHT:__________   SLEEP:__________   CALORIES:__________

EXERCISES	SETS	REPS	WT	REST	TIME	1 RM	NOTES

DATE:__________   WEIGHT:__________   SLEEP:__________   CALORIES:__________

EXERCISES	SETS	REPS	WT	REST	TIME	1 RM	NOTES

DATE:__________   WEIGHT:__________   SLEEP:__________   CALORIES:__________

EXERCISES	SETS	REPS	WT	REST	TIME	1 RM	NOTES

DATE:__________   WEIGHT:__________   SLEEP:__________   CALORIES:__________

WORKOUT LOG

NAME:____________________________ GOALS:____________________________

EXERCISES	SETS	REPS	WT	REST	TIME	1 RM	NOTES

DATE:__________ WEIGHT:__________ SLEEP:__________ CALORIES:__________

EXERCISES	SETS	REPS	WT	REST	TIME	1 RM	NOTES

DATE:__________ WEIGHT:__________ SLEEP:__________ CALORIES:__________

EXERCISES	SETS	REPS	WT	REST	TIME	1 RM	NOTES

DATE:__________ WEIGHT:__________ SLEEP:__________ CALORIES:__________

EXERCISES	SETS	REPS	WT	REST	TIME	1 RM	NOTES

DATE:__________ WEIGHT:__________ SLEEP:__________ CALORIES:__________

EXERCISES	SETS	REPS	WT	REST	TIME	1 RM	NOTES

DATE:__________ WEIGHT:__________ SLEEP:__________ CALORIES:__________

WORKOUT LOG

NAME:______________________________   GOALS:______________________________

EXERCISES	SETS	REPS	WT	REST	TIME	1 RM	NOTES

DATE:__________   WEIGHT:__________   SLEEP:__________   CALORIES:__________

EXERCISES	SETS	REPS	WT	REST	TIME	1 RM	NOTES

DATE:__________   WEIGHT:__________   SLEEP:__________   CALORIES:__________

EXERCISES	SETS	REPS	WT	REST	TIME	1 RM	NOTES

DATE:__________   WEIGHT:__________   SLEEP:__________   CALORIES:__________

EXERCISES	SETS	REPS	WT	REST	TIME	1 RM	NOTES

DATE:__________   WEIGHT:__________   SLEEP:__________   CALORIES:__________

EXERCISES	SETS	REPS	WT	REST	TIME	1 RM	NOTES

DATE:__________   WEIGHT:__________   SLEEP:__________   CALORIES:__________

WORKOUT LOG

NAME:_________________________ GOALS:_____________________________

EXERCISES	SETS	REPS	WT	REST	TIME	1 RM	NOTES

DATE:__________ WEIGHT:__________ SLEEP:__________ CALORIES:__________

EXERCISES	SETS	REPS	WT	REST	TIME	1 RM	NOTES

DATE:__________ WEIGHT:__________ SLEEP:__________ CALORIES:__________

EXERCISES	SETS	REPS	WT	REST	TIME	1 RM	NOTES

DATE:__________ WEIGHT:__________ SLEEP:__________ CALORIES:__________

EXERCISES	SETS	REPS	WT	REST	TIME	1 RM	NOTES

DATE:__________ WEIGHT:__________ SLEEP:__________ CALORIES:__________

EXERCISES	SETS	REPS	WT	REST	TIME	1 RM	NOTES

DATE:__________ WEIGHT:__________ SLEEP:__________ CALORIES:__________

WORKOUT LOG

NAME:_________________________ GOALS:_________________________

EXERCISES	SETS	REPS	WT	REST	TIME	1 RM	NOTES

DATE:_________ WEIGHT:_________ SLEEP:_________ CALORIES:_________

EXERCISES	SETS	REPS	WT	REST	TIME	1 RM	NOTES

DATE:_________ WEIGHT:_________ SLEEP:_________ CALORIES:_________

EXERCISES	SETS	REPS	WT	REST	TIME	1 RM	NOTES

DATE:_________ WEIGHT:_________ SLEEP:_________ CALORIES:_________

EXERCISES	SETS	REPS	WT	REST	TIME	1 RM	NOTES

DATE:_________ WEIGHT:_________ SLEEP:_________ CALORIES:_________

EXERCISES	SETS	REPS	WT	REST	TIME	1 RM	NOTES

DATE:_________ WEIGHT:_________ SLEEP:_________ CALORIES:_________

WORKOUT LOG

NAME:____________________ GOALS:____________________

EXERCISES	SETS	REPS	WT	REST	TIME	1 RM	NOTES

DATE:__________ WEIGHT:__________ SLEEP:__________ CALORIES:__________

EXERCISES	SETS	REPS	WT	REST	TIME	1 RM	NOTES

DATE:__________ WEIGHT:__________ SLEEP:__________ CALORIES:__________

EXERCISES	SETS	REPS	WT	REST	TIME	1 RM	NOTES

DATE:__________ WEIGHT:__________ SLEEP:__________ CALORIES:__________

EXERCISES	SETS	REPS	WT	REST	TIME	1 RM	NOTES

DATE:__________ WEIGHT:__________ SLEEP:__________ CALORIES:__________

EXERCISES	SETS	REPS	WT	REST	TIME	1 RM	NOTES

DATE:__________ WEIGHT:__________ SLEEP:__________ CALORIES:__________

WORKOUT LOG

NAME:________________________   GOALS:________________________

EXERCISES	SETS	REPS	WT	REST	TIME	1 RM	NOTES

DATE:__________   WEIGHT:__________   SLEEP:__________   CALORIES:__________

EXERCISES	SETS	REPS	WT	REST	TIME	1 RM	NOTES

DATE:__________   WEIGHT:__________   SLEEP:__________   CALORIES:__________

EXERCISES	SETS	REPS	WT	REST	TIME	1 RM	NOTES

DATE:__________   WEIGHT:__________   SLEEP:__________   CALORIES:__________

EXERCISES	SETS	REPS	WT	REST	TIME	1 RM	NOTES

DATE:__________   WEIGHT:__________   SLEEP:__________   CALORIES:__________

EXERCISES	SETS	REPS	WT	REST	TIME	1 RM	NOTES

DATE:__________   WEIGHT:__________   SLEEP:__________   CALORIES:__________

WORKOUT LOG

NAME:________________________   GOALS:__________________________

EXERCISES	SETS	REPS	WT	REST	TIME	1 RM	NOTES

DATE:__________   WEIGHT:__________   SLEEP:__________   CALORIES:__________

EXERCISES	SETS	REPS	WT	REST	TIME	1 RM	NOTES

DATE:__________   WEIGHT:__________   SLEEP:__________   CALORIES:__________

EXERCISES	SETS	REPS	WT	REST	TIME	1 RM	NOTES

DATE:__________   WEIGHT:__________   SLEEP:__________   CALORIES:__________

EXERCISES	SETS	REPS	WT	REST	TIME	1 RM	NOTES

DATE:__________   WEIGHT:__________   SLEEP:__________   CALORIES:__________

EXERCISES	SETS	REPS	WT	REST	TIME	1 RM	NOTES

DATE:__________   WEIGHT:__________   SLEEP:__________   CALORIES:__________

WORKOUT LOG

NAME:_________________________   GOALS:_________________________

EXERCISES	SETS	REPS	WT	REST	TIME	1 RM	NOTES

DATE:_________   WEIGHT:_________   SLEEP:_________   CALORIES:_________

EXERCISES	SETS	REPS	WT	REST	TIME	1 RM	NOTES

DATE:_________   WEIGHT:_________   SLEEP:_________   CALORIES:_________

EXERCISES	SETS	REPS	WT	REST	TIME	1 RM	NOTES

DATE:_________   WEIGHT:_________   SLEEP:_________   CALORIES:_________

EXERCISES	SETS	REPS	WT	REST	TIME	1 RM	NOTES

DATE:_________   WEIGHT:_________   SLEEP:_________   CALORIES:_________

EXERCISES	SETS	REPS	WT	REST	TIME	1 RM	NOTES

DATE:_________   WEIGHT:_________   SLEEP:_________   CALORIES:_________

WORKOUT LOG

NAME:_________________________   GOALS:_________________________

EXERCISES	SETS	REPS	WT	REST	TIME	1 RM	NOTES

DATE:__________   WEIGHT:__________   SLEEP:__________   CALORIES:__________

EXERCISES	SETS	REPS	WT	REST	TIME	1 RM	NOTES

DATE:__________   WEIGHT:__________   SLEEP:__________   CALORIES:__________

EXERCISES	SETS	REPS	WT	REST	TIME	1 RM	NOTES

DATE:__________   WEIGHT:__________   SLEEP:__________   CALORIES:__________

EXERCISES	SETS	REPS	WT	REST	TIME	1 RM	NOTES

DATE:__________   WEIGHT:__________   SLEEP:__________   CALORIES:__________

EXERCISES	SETS	REPS	WT	REST	TIME	1 RM	NOTES

DATE:__________   WEIGHT:__________   SLEEP:__________   CALORIES:__________

WORKOUT LOG

NAME:_________________________ GOALS:_________________________

EXERCISES	SETS	REPS	WT	REST	TIME	1 RM	NOTES

DATE:__________ WEIGHT:__________ SLEEP:__________ CALORIES:__________

EXERCISES	SETS	REPS	WT	REST	TIME	1 RM	NOTES

DATE:__________ WEIGHT:__________ SLEEP:__________ CALORIES:__________

EXERCISES	SETS	REPS	WT	REST	TIME	1 RM	NOTES

DATE:__________ WEIGHT:__________ SLEEP:__________ CALORIES:__________

EXERCISES	SETS	REPS	WT	REST	TIME	1 RM	NOTES

DATE:__________ WEIGHT:__________ SLEEP:__________ CALORIES:__________

EXERCISES	SETS	REPS	WT	REST	TIME	1 RM	NOTES

DATE:__________ WEIGHT:__________ SLEEP:__________ CALORIES:__________

WORKOUT LOG

NAME:__________________________ GOALS:__________________________

EXERCISES	SETS	REPS	WT	REST	TIME	1 RM	NOTES

DATE:__________ WEIGHT:__________ SLEEP:__________ CALORIES:__________

EXERCISES	SETS	REPS	WT	REST	TIME	1 RM	NOTES

DATE:__________ WEIGHT:__________ SLEEP:__________ CALORIES:__________

EXERCISES	SETS	REPS	WT	REST	TIME	1 RM	NOTES

DATE:__________ WEIGHT:__________ SLEEP:__________ CALORIES:__________

EXERCISES	SETS	REPS	WT	REST	TIME	1 RM	NOTES

DATE:__________ WEIGHT:__________ SLEEP:__________ CALORIES:__________

EXERCISES	SETS	REPS	WT	REST	TIME	1 RM	NOTES

DATE:__________ WEIGHT:__________ SLEEP:__________ CALORIES:__________

WORKOUT LOG

NAME:______________________________ GOALS:______________________________

EXERCISES	SETS	REPS	WT	REST	TIME	1 RM	NOTES

DATE:__________ WEIGHT:__________ SLEEP:__________ CALORIES:__________

EXERCISES	SETS	REPS	WT	REST	TIME	1 RM	NOTES

DATE:__________ WEIGHT:__________ SLEEP:__________ CALORIES:__________

EXERCISES	SETS	REPS	WT	REST	TIME	1 RM	NOTES

DATE:__________ WEIGHT:__________ SLEEP:__________ CALORIES:__________

EXERCISES	SETS	REPS	WT	REST	TIME	1 RM	NOTES

DATE:__________ WEIGHT:__________ SLEEP:__________ CALORIES:__________

EXERCISES	SETS	REPS	WT	REST	TIME	1 RM	NOTES

DATE:__________ WEIGHT:__________ SLEEP:__________ CALORIES:__________

www.ingramcontent.com/pod-product-compliance
Lightning Source LLC
Chambersburg PA
CBHW070738250726
48662CB00004B/1576